P9-ELU-903

Dr. Earl Mindell's

What You Should Know About Creating Your Personal Vitamin Plan

Other books by Dr. Earl Mindell

Dr. Earl Mindell's Garlic: The Miracle Nutrient
Dr. Earl Mindell's Live Longer & Feel Better
With Vitamins & Minerals

Dr. Earl Mindell's

What You Should Know About Creating Your Personal Vitamin Plan

Earl L. Mindell, R.Ph., Ph.D.

with Virginia L. Hopkins

Keats Publishing, Inc.　　New Canaan, Connecticut

Dr. Earl Mindell's What You Should Know About Creating Your Personal Vitamin Plan is intended solely for informational and educational purposes, and not as medical advice. Please consult a medical or health professional if you have questions about your health.

DR. EARL MINDELL'S WHAT YOU SHOULD KNOW ABOUT CREATING YOUR PERSONAL VITAMIN PLAN

Copyright © 1996 by Earl L. Mindell

All Rights Reserved

No part of this book may be reproduced in any form without the written consent of the publisher.

Library of Congress Cataloging-in-Publication Data

Mindell, Earl.
  [What you should know about creating your personal vitamin plan]
  Dr. Earl Mindell's what you should know about creating your personla vitamin plan / by Earl Mindell with Virginia L. Hopkins.
      p. cm.
  Includes bibliographical references and index.
  ISBN 0-87983-7846-2
  1. Vitamins in human nutrition—Popular works. I. Hopkins, Virginia. II. Title.
RA784.M515 1996
513.2'8—dc20   96-638
                                                        CIP

Printed in the United States of America

Keats Publishing, Inc.
27 Pine Street (Box 876)
New Canaan, Connecticut 06840-0876

99 98 97 96 6   5 4 3 2 1

CONTENTS

PART I
Getting Acquainted with Your Supplements

CHAPTER 1

The ABC's of Supplements

Entering a store that specializes in selling supplements can be an overwhelming experience for someone who doesn't know their ABC's—that's vitamin A, vitamin B and vitamin C! This book is designed to give you a basic overview of what I consider to be your essential daily supplements, including vitamins, minerals, amino acids and antioxidants. You'll also find individual vitamin plans for your age, sex and lifestyle, as well as plenty of information about treating specific health concerns with nutritional supplements.

You'll notice that all of the supplement amounts I recommend are higher than the RDA (Recommended Dietary Allowance) set by the government. This is because the RDA is the amount of the vitamin you need to take to keep you from getting a vitamin deficiency disease. This is a long way from the amount of vitamins you need to keep you in great health for the rest of your life!

If you start with my basic vitamin plan and adapt to your own personal needs, you'll be well on your way to a life of optimal health and energy. For more details on any of the topics in this book, you can refer to the long list of other books I've written in the back of this book.

DO I REALLY NEED TO TAKE VITAMINS?

If you were to eat the best possible diet of nutrient-rich organic foods, and live a stress-free life, and your environment was free of pollutants and toxins, you would not need vitamins. The reality of our lives is much different. It is virtually impossible to escape the pervasive pollution of our environment. Our soil is depleted of many essential minerals, and by the time once-fresh fruits and vegetables reach us in the super-market, they have lost much of their nutritional value. We eat processed foods and junk foods with little or no nutritional value, and we eat dozens of pounds of sugar and salt per year more than is good for us. Add to that the stresses of daily life, prescription drugs, exposure to estrogenic hormones in meat, and all the other factors in our daily lives that pull our biochemis-try out of balance, and the need for vitamins becomes apparent. In today's world, we need to take supple-ments just to maintain our health and prevent the onset of chronic diseases.

Taking vitamins and other supplements is health insurance that makes up for what you're not getting in your diet, and for the added nutritional demands made on the body by stressful lifestyles. Illness, aging and genetic weaknesses add to your individual nutri-tional needs. If there is a lot of cancer in your immedi-ate family, you should be taking the supplements that are known to help prevent cancer, such as vitamin E and selenium. If your family has a history of heart disease, you need to create a heart-healthy lifestyle that includes a low-fat diet, plenty of exercise, and plenty of antioxidants and magnesium.

The key to creating your own individual vitamin plan is paying attention to your body's needs. If you find you're getting colds a lot, there are lifestyle fac-tors you'll want to evaluate, such as whether you're getting enough sleep, whether you're allergic to some-thing in your diet or something in your home or of-fice, or maybe simply whether you're dressing warmly enough in cold weather. But you'll also want to increase your vitamin C consumption, your vitamin E consumption, and possibly your zinc (and you may want to take the useful herb echinacea) at the first sign of the sniffles.

Taking vitamins is not a substitute for a good diet or a healthy lifestyle. A vitamin can never reproduce all the nutrition packed into a fresh vegetable, or an egg, for example. The single biggest factor that shows up in studies of heart disease, cancer and aging over and over again, is that those who eat the most fresh vegetables live the longest, healthiest lives. And no amount of antioxidants will substitute for drinking plenty of clean water and moderate exercise. Nonetheless, taking vitamins is your backup plan for good health, providing the extra support you need to go beyond simply maintaining your health to having lots of energy and a clear mind.

FOR BEST RESULTS . . .

Most vitamins and minerals are best absorbed when taken with other foods, spaced out as evenly as possible during the day. The best time to take supplements is after meals. The amino acids are an exception to this. If you are taking a separate amino acid supplement, it is usually best to take it between meals.

Since some vitamins can be excreted in the urine, taking your vitamins after breakfast, after lunch and after dinner will give you the highest body level of nutrients. If you must take your vitamins all at one time, taking them after the largest meal of the day will usually give the best results.

Minerals and vitamins are mutually dependent upon each other for proper absorption. For example, vitamin C aids in the absorption of iron. Calcium aids in the absorption of vitamin D, and zinc aids in the absorption of vitamin A. So take your minerals and vitamins together.

TABLETS, CAPSULES AND LIQUIDS

Supplements come in many forms, but the most common are tablets, capsules and liquids. Multivitamins generally come in tablet form, but be sure they aren't so large you can't swallow them, and that they actually dissolve once they get to your digestive system. One way to find out how well vitamin tablets dissolve is to drop one in a little bit of vinegar, which approximates the acidity of your stomach. Depending on its size, the tablet should be nearly completely dissolved within an hour. If it isn't, you can bet you're not getting the full value from it. Some supplements work best in the small intestine, and these may be put into a tablet with a special coating that doesn't allow it to dissolve until it is out of the stomach.

Capsules are usually gelatin shells filled with the powdered form of the supplement. The gelatin dissolves quickly in the stomach, allowing the supplement to begin its work right away.

If you have trouble absorbing nutrients, you may want to consider some of the powdered or liquid vitamins, which don't have to be broken down as much in the gut.

CHAPTER 2

Vitamins Everyone Should Take Every Day

There are some vitamins that everyone, regardless of age or lifestyle, should take every day. These vitamins are essential for good health and peak energy, as they have a great many jobs to do in the body.

VITAMIN A /BETA-CAROTENE

Vitamin A is a fat-soluble vitamin that is stored in your body and doesn't need to be supplemented daily except in relatively small amounts. In fact, taking vitamin A in large doses over a long period of time can cause a toxic reaction because it accumulates in the body.

Vitamin A promotes growth, strong bones, healthy skin, is essential to the production of sex hormones, and works closely with zinc. People with acne can often eradicate it just by taking a vitamin A supplement for a few months. Vitamin A is also known as an anti-infective because it can help fight infections. In fact, if you have any type of lung infection, taking an extra vitamin A supplement for a week or two can help knock it out. Vitamin A is also called the ophthalmic vitamin because it helps improve eyesight.

Vitamin A is found in many vegetables, especially the orange and yellow vegetables such as carrots, squash, yams and cantaloupe. It's also found in liver, fish oil and eggs. One carrot can deliver up to 15,000

International Units of beta-carotene. Add a carrot a day to your apple a day!

Beta-carotene is a precursor to vitamin A, meaning that the body can make vitamin A from beta-carotene. That's the best way to get your vitamin A in a supplement, because it doesn't accumulate in the body the way vitamin A does. Beta-carotene is a potent antioxidant. Many recent studies have shown that people who have plenty of beta-carotene in their diet have a lower rate of cancer and coronary artery disease.

THE B-COMPLEX VITAMINS

The B-complex family are water-soluble vitamins involved in nearly every function of the body, from the manufacture of sex hormones and the health of brain neurons, to breaking down food and forming healthy red blood cells. The B vitamins play a key role in converting carbohydrate foods into glucose, or simple sugars, for use as energy.

The B-complex vitamins I'm going to cover here include vitamin B_1 (thiamine), vitamin B_2 (riboflavin), vitamin B_3 (niacin), vitamin B_6 (pyridoxine), vitamin B_{12} (cyanocobalamin), biotin, folic acid, inositol and vitamin B_5 (calcium pantothenate). It's best to take the B-complex vitamins together, because too much or too little of one can throw the others out of balance.

The B vitamins are found in whole grains, many nuts and root vegetables, meat, poultry, fish, eggs, dairy products and fruit.

VITAMIN B_1/Thiamine

Vitamin B_1 promotes growth, aids in the digestion of carbohydrates, can improve your mental attitude, can help fight sea and air sickness, relieves dental postoperative pain, and aids in the treatment of shingles and other herpes viruses. Vitamin B_1 is also essential for normal functioning of nerve tissues, muscles and heart. Taking vitamin B_1 as a supplement can create an odor on the skin that humans can't smell, but that repels insects, especially mosquitoes.

Smokers, drinkers, heavy sugar consumers, antacid users and those on birth control pills need more B_1.

Vitamin B_1 can cause high blood pressure in excess.

VITAMIN B_2/Riboflavin

Vitamin B_2 aids in growth and reproduction, promotes healthy hair, skin and nails, alleviates eye fatigue, eliminates sore mouth and lips, helps your body burn carbohydrates, fats and proteins. A deficiency of vitamin B_2 may cause a decreased ability to generate antibodies, which help the body resist disease. A deficiency may also result in itching and burning of the eyes, cracking of the corners of the lips, and inflammation of the mouth. If you are a heavy coffee or alcohol drinker, on the Pill, under a lot of stress, or eat lots of processed foods (please don't!), you may need extra vitamin B_2. Natural sources of vitamin B_2 include liver, kidney, milk, cheese, and most B_1 sources.

VITAMIN B_3/Niacin/niacinamide

Niacin is the most potent and effective cholesterol-lowering substance known. The only reason it isn't the best-selling cholesterol-lowering medicine is because it's an inexpensive, natural substance that can't be patented by the drug companies. If they can't patent it, they can't charge you high prices, so they aren't interested in promoting it. Niacin not only lowers LDL or "bad" cholesterol, it also raises HDL or "good" cholesterol. (If your physician has you on cholesterol-lowering drugs, don't stop taking them without supervision.)

Niacin has gotten some bad press. Some forms of it can cause flushing and itching, and high prolonged doses of timed-release niacin can cause liver problems. If you begin with a small dose and gradually work your way up to a higher dose, you should be able to minimize these problems. Niacinamide is more often used than niacin, since it minimizes the burning, flushing and itching of the skin that frequently occurs with nicotinic acid. More recently, some vitamin manufacturers have developed "no-flush" niacin formulas that deliver all of the benefits of niacin without the unpleasant side effects. These formulas are made by combining niacin with inositol hexanicotinate, an ester involved in sending messages within the nervous system. In any case, niacin is still safer and more effective than any of the pharmaceutical cholesterol-lowering drugs.

Niacin also aids in promoting a healthy digestive system, gives you healthy skin, can prevent or ease the severity of migraine headaches, increases circulation, especially in the upper body, can reduce high blood pressure, is an antidiarrheal, increases your energy through proper food utilization, helps fight canker sores, helps fight bad breath, is a possible cancer inhibitor, and is necessary for the metabolism of sugar.

Niacin is found naturally in lean meat, whole grains, green vegetables, and beans.

VITAMIN B₆/Pyridoxine

This vitamin is actually a group of vitamins called pyridoxine, pyridoxal and pyridoxamine, but B₆ is often just called pyridoxine. This important vitamin is crucial to the formation of all the steroid hormones, including the sex hormones and the cortisones. Women can often correct PMS and menopause problems simply by taking a vitamin B₆ supplement. It also helps protect against osteoporosis. This B vitamin also plays an essential role in maintaining a healthy nervous system and a healthy cardiovascular system. Researchers have recently recognized that a high level of homocysteine, a by-product of amino acid metabolism, is at least as important a risk factor in heart disease as high cholesterol or high blood pressure, and vitamin B_6, together with the B vitamins folic acid and vitamin B_{12}, reduces the level of homocysteine in the body.

Vitamin B_6 also helps assimilate protein and fat, aids in converting tryptophan to niacin, is an antinauseant (effective for morning sickness), can help with PMS and menopause symptoms, helps synthesize antiaging nucleic acids, reduces "cotton mouth" and urination problems caused by tricyclic antidepressant drugs, reduces night muscle spasms, leg cramps and hand numbness, and works as a natural diuretic. If you want to know more about vitamin B_6, I highly recommend Dr. Alan Gaby's book on the subject, *The Doctor's Guide to Vitamin B_6* (Rodale Press, 1984).

Vitamin B_6 occurs naturally in meat, fish, egg yolk, cantaloupe, cabbage, milk, soy products, peanuts, and brown rice.

A deficiency of vitamin B_6 may result in nervousness, insomnia, skin eruptions and loss of muscular control.

Vitamin B_6 can be toxic in high doses. Please don't take over 500 mg a day.

VITAMIN B_{12}/Cobalamin

Vitamin B_{12} is commonly known as the "red vitamin," cobalamin. Since it is so effective in small doses, it is one of the few vitamins generally recommended in microgram (mcg) doses. Vitamin B_{12} is not well absorbed in the digestive tract, so the best ways to take it in are intranasally or sublingually (under the tongue).

I believe that a very high percentage of senility

symptoms in older people are caused by a simple vitamin B_{12} and folic acid deficiency. As we age, we don't produce as much stomach acid and as a result we don't absorb our food as well. This is particularly true of the B vitamins, and especially B_{12}. Many older people tend to have poor nutrition anyway, but even with good nutrition, if there is an absorption problem, a vitamin B_{12} deficiency may result. Anyone over the age of 50 who is experiencing problems such as memory loss, forgetfulness, depression, loss of appetite, and fatigue, should try a few weeks of B_{12} shots (given by doctors and other health care professionals) to see if the symptoms clear up. Supplements of folic acid and vitamin B_6 should be given along with the B_{12}, as they work best together.

Vitamin B_{12} also forms and regenerates red blood cells which carry oxygen to the tissues, giving you more energy and preventing anemia, promotes growth and gives children an increased appetite, is important for maintenance of a healthy nervous system, can relieve irritability, improves circulation, memory, and balance, and can enhance immunity in the elderly. Vitamin B_{12} also plays an important role, along with folic acid and vitamin B_6, in keeping homocysteine levels low. As I mentioned earlier, homocysteine raises the risk of heart disease.

Vitamin B_{12} is found naturally in liver, beef, pork, eggs, milk, cheese. Vitamin B_{12} is only found in animal foods in significant amounts, so if you are a vegetarian it is important to take a B_{12} supplement.

BIOTIN

Biotin is one of the more recently discovered B vitamins, but it is a key vitamin in maintaining healthy hair and skin. It can keep your hair from turning gray, prevent baldness, ease muscle pains, and is important for healthy skin.

Biotin is found naturally in whole grains, milk, vegetables and nuts. It is present in minute quantities in every living cell and is also synthesized by intestinal bacteria.

A deficiency of biotin may lead to hair loss, extreme exhaustion, drowsiness, muscle pains and loss of appetite.

CHOLINE

Choline is an ingredient in lecithin, a naturally-occurring fat emulsifier found in eggs, soy and other legumes, nuts and some meats such as liver. Choline is one of the few substances able to penetrate the blood-brain barrier, going directly to brain cells, where it plays a role in transmitting nerve impulses. For this reason, taking lecithin may help with memory, ability to learn, symptoms of senility and Alzheimer's.

Because of its effects on fats, choline can lower cholesterol, aids the liver in removing poisons and drugs from your bloodstream, is necessary for normal fat metabolism, and minimizes excessive deposits of fat in liver.

Lecithin and choline are found naturally in egg yolks, green leafy vegetables and legumes.

A deficiency of choline may result in cirrhosis and fatty degeneration of the liver, and hardening of the arteries.

FOLIC ACID

Folic acid has recently been recognized as a key vitamin in preventing a type of birth defect called neural tube defects, such as spina bifida. It is important that all sexually active women at any risk whatsoever for getting pregnant get at least 200 mcg of folic acid every day, and preferably 400 mcg.

Folic acid also works hand in hand with vitamin B_6 and vitamin B_{12} to reduce the levels of harmful homocysteine in the blood. A deficiency of folic acid, vitamin B_6 and vitamin B_{12} significantly raises your risk of heart disease by raising homocysteine levels.

Folic acid also improves lactation in nursing women, can act as a pain reliever, delays gray hair (along with PABA and pantothenic acid), prevents canker sores, helps against anemia (along with iron, copper and vitamin C), is essential to the formation of red blood cells by its action on the bone marrow, aids in protein metabolism, and contributes to normal growth.

Too much folic acid can cause problems for epileptics and people with allergies.

Folic acid is found naturally in deep green leafy vegetables, and meat.

INOSITOL

Inositol combines with choline to form lecithin, and has many of the same benefits. It can be very helpful in treating eczema. It also lowers cholesterol, is important for healthy hair, helps metabolize body fat, is a relaxant, and can help relieve diabetic peripheral neuropathy.

Inositol is found naturally in fruits, nuts, whole grains, milk, and meat. Cantaloupe and citrus fruits are especially good sources.

VITAMIN B₅/Calcium Pantothenate

Calcium pantothenate is also called pantothenic acid. It is involved in the growth of cells, helps maintain normal skin, is crucial to the development of the central nervous system, is required for synthesis of antibodies, is necessary for normal digestive processes, helps heal wounds, prevents fatigue, is an antiallergy and stress supplement, and fights infections. In some people calcium pantothenate helps relieve arthritis symptoms, but in other people it can aggravate them.

Calcium pantothenate is found naturally in organ meats, eggs, whole grains, bran, peas.

VITAMIN C

Vitamin C, also called ascorbic acid, is water-soluble, and one of the superstars of the vitamin world. It is a powerful antioxidant that slows the aging process and helps prevent heart disease and cancer. It also plays an important role in healing wounds, helps prevent fatigue, is an antihistamine, helping to reduce allergy symptoms, helps fight infections by building antibodies, can stop bleeding gums, lowers cholesterol, is an anticancer agent, prevents the production of nitrosamines (cancer-causing agents), is a natural laxative, lowers the incidence of blood clots in the veins, therefore decreasing the risk of heart attack and stroke, decreases the severity and length of the common cold, and increases the absorption of iron. Vitamin C works as a team with other vitamins, minerals and enzymes, strengthening the collagen in connective tissue and promoting capillary integrity.

Vitamin C is found naturally in nearly all fresh foods and meat. It is especially high in citrus fruits, berries, greens, cabbages and peppers. Vitamin C is destroyed by cooking, which is one of the many reasons it is important to eat plenty of fresh, raw fruits and vegetables.

Vitamin C in large doses can cause mild diarrhea. Either buy an esterfied form of vitamin C, or back off the dose until the diarrhea stops.

VITAMIN D

Vitamin D is also called calciferous, ergosterol, and the "sunshine vitamin." This hormonelike vitamin regulates the use of calcium and phosphorus in the body and is therefore necessary for the proper formation of teeth and bones. It is especially important in infancy and childhood. Most of our vitamin D is manufactured in the body when our skin is exposed to sunlight. This is why it's important to get regular sun. Taken with A and C, vitamin D can help to prevent colds. It is also used to treat conjunctivitis.

Vitamin D is also found naturally in fish oil, fat, and dairy products. Vitamin D should not be taken in high doses long term because it accumulates in the body and can be toxic at high doses. However, it can be an essential vitamin for people who aren't getting outdoors in the sun.

VITAMIN E

Vitamin E is also called tocopherol. It is available in several different forms, both as a liquid and solid. Vitamin E is another superstar in the vitamin world, able to help us fend off heart disease and important to hundreds of biochemical processes in the body. Vitamin E is a powerful antioxidant that slows the aging process and also helps prevent cancer. It works with beta-carotene to protect the lungs from pollution, prevents and dissolves blood clots, helps prevent scarring when used externally on the skin, accelerates burn healing, can lower blood pressure by its diuretic action, prevents night cramps, lazy leg and leg cramps, helps prevent cataracts, and enhances the immune system.

Vitamin E is found naturally in whole grains,

green leafy vegetables, vegetable oils, meat, eggs, and avocados.

Today many cardiologists recommend 400 IU of Vitamin E daily. The dry (succinate) form of Vitamin E is preferred for people over 40 because it is more easily absorbed by the digestive system.

BIOFLAVONOIDS

Bioflavonoids are organic compounds found in plants. These powerful substances reduce inflammation and pain, strengthen blood vessels, improve circulation, fight bacteria and viruses, improve liver function, lower cholesterol levels and improve vision. Bioflavonoids help prevent bruising by strengthening capillary walls. For this reason, they are also helpful for diabetics in improving circulation, and can help prevent eye problems such as cataracts and macular degeneration. Bioflavonoids are also beneficial in hypertension, and help build resistance to infections and colds.

Vitamin C is found combined with bioflavonoids in nature, and in supplements works much more effectively when combined with bioflavonoids.

Bioflavonoids are found in a wide variety of plants. Some of the best food sources are the white material underneath citrus fruit peels, peppers, and berries. Although bioflavonoids are not considered essential to life, and therefore are not classified as vitamins, it is becoming clear that they *are* essential to good health.

Whatever vitamin C you are taking should be combined with a bioflavonoid complex. Each works best when combined with the other.

CHAPTER 3

Minerals Everyone Should Take Every Day

Minerals work in partnership with hormones, enzymes, amino acids and vitamins. They are required to build and maintain the structure of the body. They are involved in the breakdown of food during digestion, and some are instrumental in maintaining fluid balance inside cells. Those that are currently considered essential for human nutrition are: calcium, phosphorus, iron, potassium, selenium, magnesium and zinc. In reality however, many more minerals are needed to maintain optimal health. Chromium, cobalt, copper, manganese and potassium are important in their own right, even though we only require them in very small amounts.

Processed or refined foods (for example: white flour and white sugar) are almost devoid of minerals, which is one reason I strongly recommend eating whole foods such as grains, fruits and vegetables, which are very rich in minerals in their unrefined state.

Another reason we tend to be deficient in minerals is that our soil is depleted. Modern agricultural methods using commercial fertilizers do not replace the rich array of minerals found naturally in soil, so vegetables grown in those soils do not have the minerals we need for good health. This is one of the best reasons I know of to eat organic fruits and vegetables (besides reducing your exposure to pesticides).

Unless you are trying to correct a specific nutritional deficiency under the supervision of a health-care professional, minerals should only be taken in the recommended doses. An excess of minerals can cause just as many problems as a deficiency.

Let's take a closer look at the minerals you should be getting in your daily vitamin program.

CALCIUM

Calcium is the most abundant mineral in the body. It builds and maintains bones and teeth, helps blood to clot, aids vitality and endurance, regulates heart rhythm and helps muscles relax. Calcium also plays a role in maintaining fluid balance within the cells. Calcium can't do its work maintaining strong bones without its partners magnesium and phosphorus. Most of us get plenty of phosphorus in our diets, but many North Americans are deficient in magnesium, and calcium should always be taken with magnesium. There is some disagreement about what the ratio of calcium to magnesium should be, but most supplements provide a three to one ratio of calcium to magnesium, which is fine. Because of their relaxing effect on the muscles, calcium and magnesium can be taken just before bed to aid in sleeping and to prevent leg cramps.

Contrary to popular opinion, milk is not a good source of calcium because it has a poor calcium-to-magnesium ratio, so the body can't put it to work. I believe dairy products cause more health problems than they solve, and I recommend that you get the majority of your calcium from fresh vegetables, especially leafy green vegetables, soy foods, sardines, salmon and nuts. A high protein diet and excessive consumption of phosphorus-containing sodas can deplete calcium from the bones.

BORON

Boron is a trace mineral that helps retard bone loss and works with calcium, magnesium and vitamin D to help prevent osteoporosis (brittle bones). Boron is abundant in apples and grapes.

CHROMIUM

Chromium works with insulin in the metabolism of sugar and helps the body utilize protein and fats. Taken in conjunction with exercise, chromium helps the body burn off fat more efficiently. It is best to take chromium in the form of chromium picolinate. Chromium also helps prevent and lower high blood pressure.

COBALT

Cobalt is a stimulant to the production of red blood cells, is a component of vitamin B_{12}, and is necessary for normal growth. A deficiency of cobalt can cause anemia.

COPPER

Copper and zinc balance each other in the body, and a deficiency of one can cause an excess of the other. Copper is necessary for absorption and utilization of iron and the formation of red blood cells.

IRON

Iron is required in manufacture of hemoglobin, a component of blood, and helps carry oxygen in the blood. It works with many enzymes in biochemical reactions in the body, and to be used efficiently must also have copper, cobalt, manganese and vitamin C.

Iron is not efficiently excreted from the body, and can accumulate in tissues. Recent research has shown that excessive amounts of iron in the tissues raise the risk of heart disease. Some researchers theorize that part of the reason a woman's risk of heart disease increases after menopause is that she is not losing iron every month during menstruation. Although iron is an essential mineral, it is important not to take too much iron in supplement form. A deficiency can cause a specific disease called iron deficiency anemia.

MAGNESIUM

Magnesium is one of the superstars of the mineral world. It is necessary for calcium and vitamin C metabolism and literally hundreds of enzyme reactions in the body. It plays a key role in regulating fluid balance in the cells, and is essential for normal functioning of the nervous, muscular and cardiovascular systems. Magnesium deficiency is very common in North America, and I believe that it is a more common and important risk factor for heart disease than mainstream medicine acknowledges. I recommend that anyone with heart disease or at risk for heart disease take an extra supplement of 300-400 mg of magnesium daily. Fatigue and muscle weakness can also be signs of magnesium deficiency.

Magnesium is found naturally in whole grains, figs, nuts and seeds, bananas and other fruits, and green vegetables.

MANGANESE

Manganese is an important trace mineral that activates various enzymes and other minerals and is related to proper utilization of vitamins B_1 and E. Manganese is also involved with thyroid function, the central nervous system and digestion.

POTASSIUM

Potassium is a key mineral in regulating the pH balance and fluid balance in the body. It balances sodium in the cells and, along with calcium and magnesium, regulates heart rhythm. Potassium can be depleted by any type of abnormally large fluid loss such as strenuous exercise, diarrhea, hypoglycemia, and the use of diuretics such as those used to lower blood pressure. When potassium is deficient, it can cause nerve and muscle dysfunction, bloating due to water retention, ringing in the ears, and insomnia. Potassium is naturally found in citrus fruits, cantaloupe, tomatoes, watercress, all green leafy vegetables, the mints, sunflower seeds, bananas and potatoes. Most people can easily get enough potassium in their daily diet, but many multivitamins contain potassium. Please don't take potassium supplements without the supervision of a health care professional, as an excess can throw other minerals out of balance and affect fluid balance in the cells.

SELENIUM

Selenium could be called the anticancer mineral. Over and over again population studies have shown that people living in geographical areas containing plenty of selenium in the soil have lower rates of cancer, and those living in areas with selenium-depleted soil have a higher rate of cancer, especially colon cancer. Selenium is an antioxidant that also stimulates the immune system. It works synergistically with vitamin E, each enhancing the actions of the other. Selenium is found in high concentrations in semen, and men seem to need more of this mineral than women. A selenium deficiency can cause dandruff, dry skin and fatigue.

ZINC

An essential mineral, zinc plays multiple roles. It controls muscle contractions, along with magnesium and calcium, helps normal tissue function, and is essential in protein and carbohydrate metabolism and the functioning of the immune system. A lack of zinc in your diet can increase fatigue and cause a susceptibility to infection and injury, as well as a reduction in alertness. When you exercise vigorously, you lose a lot of zinc, so it's important for athletes to take a zinc supplement. Zinc is found in many foods, including most vegetables, whole grains, dairy products, many nuts and seeds, fish and meat.

Zinc should be present in all good multivitamin formulas. But as with all minerals, please don't take zinc in excess, as it will cause other imbalances in your body. Zinc works best in combination with vitamin A, calcium and phosphorus.

CHAPTER 4

The Amazing Amino Acids

Protein is made up of amino acids. Although there are dozens of amino acids, only some amino acids are produced in the body. All eight of the essential amino acids are made in very small amounts by the bacteria found in the intestines, but they must also be supplied from food intake.

THE ESSENTIAL AMINO ACIDS

Lysine	Phenylalanine
Leucine	Threonine
Isoleucine	Tryptophan
Methionine	Valine

The following amino acids are essential for pregnant women for their developing fetus, and for infants: histidine, taurine and cysteine. Eric R. Braverman and Carl C. Pfeiffer, in their book *The Healing Nutrients Within,* state the following amino acids to be conditionally essential, and necessary for anyone under stress: alanine, arginine, aspartic acid, carnitine, cystine, GABA, glutamic acid, glutamine, glycine, homocysteine (toxic in high doses), hydroxyproline, proline, and serine.

Amino acids play a variety of important roles in every part of the body, including the immune system, the digestive system, metabolism, detoxification, and glucose balance. In the brain, some of the amino acids taken as supplements work very well to combat depression, enhance mood and improve sleep, while others improve memory and cognitive abilities.

When we eat proteins, they are broken down into proteins or peptides, which are proteins made of only a few amino acids, and then absorbed into the body.

TAKING AMINO ACIDS

All amino acids should be taken between meals with juice or water, and not with protein, unless they are included in a multivitamin. Since individual amino acids can have such a powerful effect on the body, I recommend that, if you're taking them to treat a specific chronic problem such as heart disease or depression, you work with a health care professional.

Many amino acids serve as precursors for others. For example, cysteine is a precursor to glutathione, and since glutathione is somewhat unstable in supplement form, you can take cysteine or N-acetyl cysteine as a supplement to boost your glutathione levels.

If you're taking amino acids, taking a B-vitamin complex at the same time will enhance their absorption and metabolism.

Here is a complete list of all of the amino acids, grouped by their molecular structure and function in the body, as delineated by Braverman and Pfeiffer. If you want to know more about amino acids, I highly recommend their book.

Aromatic amino acids
Phenylalanine
Tyrosine
Tryptophan

Sulfur amino Acids
Cysteine and Glutathione
Taurine

Methionine
Homocysteine

Urea cycle amino acids
Arginine and citrulline
Ornithine

Glutamate amino acids
Glutamic acid, GABA and glutamine
Proline and hydroxyproline
Aspartic acid–asparagine

Threonine amino acids
Threonine
Glycine
Serine
Alanine

Branched chain amino acids
Leucine, isoleucine and valine

Amino acids with important metabolites
Lysine
Carnitine
Histidine

Here are some of the amino acids that should be included in vitamin regimens, especially if you are a vegetarian, aren't absorbing nutrients well, have problems with depression, or simply need a high-powered vitamin regimen:

ALANINE

Alanine is a nonessential amino acid that enhances the immune system, lowers the risk of kidney stones, and aids in alleviating hypoglycemia by regulating sugar. Alanine is released by the muscles for energy, and athletes may enhance their performance by taking alanine supplements. In very high doses alanine suppresses taurine. Alanine has also been used successfully to treat epilepsy, high cholesterol, and liver disease in alcoholics.

ARGININE

Arginine is a conditionally essential amino acid that increases sperm count in men, accelerates wound healing, tones muscle tissue, helps metabolize stored body fat, and promotes physical and mental alertness. Arginine is important in estrogen production, and a deficiency may contribute to an estrogen deficiency. Research with rodents has demonstrated that arginine can reduce the growth of tumors. Arginine can aggravate herpes and bring on an outbreak. Those who suffer from herpes outbreaks should avoid arginine supplements and arginine-containing foods such as nuts, chocolate and coffee. Arginine also should not be taken by growing children.

ASPARTIC ACID

Aspartic acid is a nonessential amino acid that is highly concentrated in the body. It can enhance the immune system, as well as increase stamina and endurance. Aspartic acid should be used as a supplement with great care because it is one of the major excitatory neurotransmitters in the brain, and can be toxic in excess. The artificial sweetener aspartame breaks down in the stomach to aspartic acid and phenylalanine (among other things), and consuming excessive amounts of these amino acids in people who are sensitive to them is related to the widespread health problems caused by aspartame, including headaches, dizziness and seizures.

CARNITINE

Although carnitine is not an essential amino acid, a deficiency can cause fatigue, muscle weakness, heart disease, acidic blood, high triglyceride levels, and brain degeneration. Taking carnitine as a supplement can enhance the body's ability to burn fat, prevent heart disease and improve brain deterioration as we age.

Lysine is a precursor to carnitine, and to manufacture carnitine, the body also needs vitamin B_6, niacin, iron, and vitamin C.

If you're at risk for heart disease, or have heart disease, carnitine is an essential supplement for you. Carnitine supplements can lower triglyceride levels, raise HDL (good) cholesterol, lower LDL (bad) cholesterol, and it improves irregular heartbeats, reduces angina attacks and has an overall strengthening effect on the heart.

Carnitine is an especially important supplement to take when you're losing weight because it cleans up substances called ketones in the blood, formed when the body is breaking down fat.

While carnitine is being used successfully to treat the symptoms of Alzheimer's and senility, you don't need to have a failing memory to benefit from it. Studies have shown that carnitine supplementation improves long term memory, increases alertness and improves learning ability and can improve mood.

Carnitine's ability to protect brain neurons and enhance their responsiveness also makes it one of our most important anti-aging supplements. Carnitine essentially acts as an antioxidant in the brain.

The forms of carnitine I recommend are either L-carnitine, acetyl L-carnitine, or L-acetylcarnitine. Please do not take the synthetic D or DL forms of carnitine, as they can have negative side effects.

CYSTINE, CYSTEINE

Cysteine is another conditionally essential amino acid and an important antiaging nutrient. Cystine and cysteine can be readily converted by the body into one another. Cysteine's most important role in the body is detoxification. In addition, it is an antioxidant. Cysteine is a precursor to the important amino acids taurine and glutathione.

When given as a supplement, cysteine raises glutathione levels in the body. Because of this, it is used routinely in hospital emergency rooms to prevent liver damage when people overdose on drugs or alcohol; to detoxify in cases of heavy metal poisoning, and is used to protect against the harmful side effects of chemotherapy and radiation. Cysteine is currently being used successfully to raise T-cell levels in AIDS patients. Cysteine is also important in preventing eye problems such as cataracts and macular degeneration.

Foods that contain high levels of cysteine include onions, garlic, yogurt, wheat germ and red meat.

A form of cysteine called N-acetyl cysteine is widely used in Europe for coughs, asthma prevention and chronic bronchitis, because it is very effective at breaking up mucus in the lungs. If you have a tendency to get a winter cough, take it at the first sign of lung troubles.

Please don't take more than the recommended dosage of cysteine, as an excess can upset the balance of your body's chemistry just as much as a deficiency can.

GAMMA-AMINOBUTYRIC ACID (GABA)

One of the best known substances that transmit nerve impulses to the brain (neurotransmitter), GABA has a calming effect. In the brain GABA balances glutamic acid, an excitatory amino acid. The three amino acids GABA, glutamic acid and glutamine are constantly being transformed into each other as needed by the body.

GABA plays a major role in brain function. The benzodiazepine drugs such as Valium work because they stimulate GABA receptors in the brain.

GABA optimizes the body's use of vitamin C, it can lower blood pressure, and it may be involved with the release of growth hormone.

GLUTAMIC ACID

Glutamic acid works closely with GABA, particularly in the brain. However, while GABA is calming, glutamic acid is the opposite, an excitatory brain amino acid. In people who are deficient in it, glutamic acid can help improve brain function, alleviate fatigue, and elevate mood. However, in excess glutamic acid can become an excitotoxin, overstimulating brain cells and killing them. I recommend you work with a health-care professional when using glutamic acid as a supplement.

GLUTAMINE

Glutamine is the third in the trio of GABA and glutamic acid. It is abundant in the brain, and in the intestines, where it plays an important role in maintaining a healthy mucous lining. Taking glutamine before and after surgery can significantly reduce healing time. Manganese is a mineral that is essential to the synthesis of glutamine, and glutamine is essential to the synthesis of niacin, as is tryptophan. Glutamine has been used successfully to help alcoholics in the withdrawal process and can greatly decrease the craving for alcohol.

Glutamine seems to be a food for cancer tumors, so please don't take this as a supplement if you have cancer. Since it plays a role in regulating brain neuro-transmitters, it can be toxic in high doses.

GLUTATHIONE

I call glutathione (known as GSH) the "triple threat" amino acid because it is a tripeptide made from the amino acids cysteine, glycine and glutamic acid. It is found in the cells of nearly all living organisms on earth, and its primary job is waste disposal. GSH has three main detox jobs in the body: 1) When there are free radicals lurking about, threatening to start an oxidation reaction, GSH catches them, neutralizes them, passes them on (often to another antioxidant such as vitamin E), and begins the cycle anew; 2) in the liver, GSH latches on to toxic substances and binds to them, so the liver can excrete them without being damaged; and 3) GSH prevents red blood cells from being damaged by neutralizing unstable forms of oxygen.

GSH also plays a role in fighting cancer, stabilizing blood sugar, and cellular repair after a stroke. Gluta-thione's antioxidant work is the front line defense for preventing oxidation of LDL cholesterol which dam-ages the arteries. It's also crucial in protecting the lymphatic system and the digestive system from an overload of unstable lipids (fats and oils). If glutathi-one levels drop anywhere in the body, the burden of toxic stress goes up.

GSH is one of the most abundant substances in the body, and as long as we have a good supply of its building block cysteine (glycine and glutamic acid are rarely in short supply) and its cofactor selenium, it will be hard at work doing its detoxifying chores. GSH levels drop as we age, and can be depleted by an over-load of rancid oils (such as polyunsaturated and par-tially hydrogenated vegetable oils), overexposure to poisons such as pesticides, and pharmaceutical drugs that stress the liver such as acetaminophen (Tylenol) and aspirin. Since glutathione often passes off its neutralized waste products to antioxidants such as vitamin C and vitamin E, a deficiency of these vitamins can impair its function.

If you have heart disease, are at a high risk for it, or have high LDL cholesterol levels, I recommend you try raising your glutathione levels. The best way to raise glutathione levels is by taking a cysteine supplement. Once again, please stick to the recommended dosage; an excess of cysteine can cause as many problems as it solves.

GLYCINE

Glycine is a conditionally essential amino acid that produces glycogen which mobilizes glucose (blood sugar) from the liver, and bolsters the immune system. Like GABA and taurine, glycine has a calming effect on the brain. A deficiency is thought to be involved with Parkinson's disease, and it may increase acetylcholine in the brain, improving memory and cognitive function.

Glycine has a sweet taste that can mask bitterness, and it is sometimes used as a sweetener. It is also used as a food additive to prevent the rancidity of fats and to act as an antioxidant. Glycine can lower cholesterol, heal gout, and speeds up wound healing. It stimulates growth hormone, and can aid in healing of a swollen and infected prostate.

HISTIDINE

Although histidine is not an essential amino acid for adults, it is an amino acid that is essential to growth, from fetal growth through infancy. It is a precursor of histamine, which stimulates inflammation in allergies.

A histidine deficiency is found in many arthritis patients, and supplementation sometimes helps. Histidine can help keep people from biting their nails, dilate blood vessels, alleviate symptoms of rheumatoid arthritis, alleviate stress, and can help increase libido. A histidine deficiency contributes to the development of cataracts. Because elevated histidine levels can cause mental problems, it is not recommended as a daily supplement for adults.

ISOLEUCINE, LEUCINE AND VALINE

Isoleucine, leucine and valine are essential amino acids known as branched chain amino acids (BCAAs). They are key ingredients in the body's ability to handle stress and produce energy. They are used by the muscles for energy, and are needed in hemoglobin formation. Taking the BCAAs as a supplement can speed healing after surgery, and may help build muscle. The BCAAs may also be brain transmitters and have some ability to relieve pain. Alcoholics and drug addicts tend to be deficient in leucine, glutamine, GABA and citrulline.

PHENYLALANINE

Phenylalanine is an essential amino acid that plays a key part in brain function and is a major precursor to many brain chemicals, including the amino acid tyrosine, and the catecholamines such as dopamine and epinephrine. Other brain chemicals such as vasopressin, somatostatin and ACTH contain phenylalanine. Morphine and codeine contain phenylalanine.

Like the other amino acids that affect brain function, phenylalanine can be very helpful as a supplement if it is deficient in some way, but can be harmful in excess. The artificial sweetener aspartame breaks down in the stomach to form aspartic acid and phenylalanine. The phenylalanine accounts for some of the adverse reactions to the sweetener. Some people are born with a sensitivity to phenylalanine called phenylketonuria (PKU). If not caught in infancy and foods containing phenylalanine avoided, PKU can cause serious retardation.

In people who are deficient in phenylalanine, it can improve memory and mental alertness, act as an antidepressant, help suppress appetite, reduce pain and increase sexual interest. It can also raise blood pressure, so be cautious in its use if you have high blood pressure. It cannot be metabolized if a person is deficient in vitamin C.

I recommend taking phenylalanine in the D or DL-phenylalanine form.

LYSINE

Lysine is an essential amino acid involved in metabolism, muscle tissue, the immune system, and growth. A deficiency may cause nausea, dizziness and anemia. Taking it as a supplement helps improve concentration, enhances fertility, aids in preventing fever blisters or cold sores (herpes simplex) and shortens the healing period for herpes. Lysine is found in meat, eggs, fish, milk and cheese. When treating a herpes outbreak, up to 5 grams (5,000 mg) a day may be taken.

METHIONINE

Methionine is an essential amino acid and plays an important role in metabolism. It is a lipotropic agent, meaning it reduces fat, particularly in the liver. It also protects the kidneys, aids in lowering cholesterol, is a natural chelating agent for heavy metals, and aids in maintaining beautiful skin. It also builds new bony tissue. A deficiency of methionine may lead to heart disease, fatty degeneration and cirrhosis of the liver.

It has been used to treat schizophrenia, Parkinson's and depression. Methionine can be found in sunflower seeds, meat, eggs, fish, milk and cheese.

PROLINE AND HYDROXYPROLINE

Proline and hydroxyproline are conditionally essential amino acids that aid in wound healing, and can help increase learning ability. These two amino acids are found in the highest amounts in the body's collagen tissue. Hydroxyproline is most important in bone and connective tissue. Proline is one of the amino acids that seems to stimulate tumor development, and people with cancer should not take it as a supplement. In fact, it is probably not necessary to supplement proline or hydroxyproline at all, as they tend to be in the body in abundance, and an excess can cause imbalances in other amino acids.

SERINE

Serine is a conditionally essential amino acid that is made from glycine and can also be made into glycine and cystine. It can help alleviate pain and produces cellular energy. An excess in the body or very high doses can cause psychosis. Serine is another amino acid that promotes tumor growth and should not be taken by anyone who has cancer. There is no need to supplement serine as our bodies tend to make what we need in abundance.

TAURINE

Taurine is an amino acid that is essential to infants but nonessential to adults. It is a very useful amino acid in treating some forms of epilepsy. It plays an important role in the heart, eyes, brain, gallbladder and blood vessels, particularly keeping fluids and mineral balance in cells stable, and stabilizing cell membranes. Taurine is an important supplement for anyone who has heart disease, but should be taken under the guidance of a health care professional if you are on heart disease drugs. Taurine is also important in stabilizing cell membranes in the brain, and is a neurotransmitter, and as such can have a calming effect. It can improve memory, and has been used to treat insomnia, anxiety and high blood pressure. The food additive MSG can reduce taurine levels. Since taurine can enhance the action of insulin, diabetics and hypoglycemics should use it with care.

THREONINE

Threonine is an essential amino acid that can be deficient in vegetarian diets. It is a precursor to the important amino acid glycine, which acts as a brain sedative. Threonine is essential to normal growth, helps prevent fatty buildup in the liver, is necessary for utilization of protein in the diet, stimulates the immune system, and has been used to treat manic depression and multiple sclerosis. A deficiency results in negative hydrogen balance in the body. Threonine levels decline with age, making them valuable antiaging supplements.

TRYPTOPHAN

Tryptophan is an essential amino acid with many valuable uses. It is a precursor to niacin, which prevents pellagra and mental deficiency. It plays a role in regulating sleep and is closely tied to the production of serotonin in the brain. A deficiency causes insomnia. It is useful as a relaxant and antianxiety agent as well.

Tryptophan was widely used as a sleep aid until a contaminated batch made in Japan reportedly killed 11 people. Unfortunately, in spite of the fact that uncontaminated tryptophan is entirely safe and is used in baby foods and nutritional powders for senior citizens, the FDA has pulled it off the market as a nutritional supplement as of this writing. Tryptophan was pulled off the market within weeks before the drug Prozac was approved by the FDA. It is interesting that the inexpensive, safe and effective tryptophan does essentially the same thing in the brain that Prozac does, without the side effects. The fact that tryptophan is not available in the US is purely political and has no basis in a lack of safety.

TYROSINE

Tyrosine is a nonessential amino acid that acts as a precursor to many other amino acids and brain chemicals. It is important in times of stress, and plays a part in maintaining a healthy thyroid gland. It also yields L-dopa, making it useful in the treatment of Parkinson's disease. It has an important role in stimulating and modifying brain activity, helps control drug resistant depression and anxiety, as well as helping amphetamine takers to reduce their dosage to minimal levels in a few weeks. It can also help cocaine addicts kick their habit, by helping to avert the depression, fatigue and extreme irritability which accompany withdrawal. It can worsen the symptoms of schizophrenia.

The artificial sweetener aspartame raises tyrosine levels in the brain, which may cause toxicity in sensitive people.

CHAPTER 5

A Few Important Antioxidants

Antioxidants are one of your best forms of health insurance, both against the modern maladies that plague so many of us, such as heart disease, cancer and diabetes, and against the diseases of aging, such as arthritis and digestive difficulties. There are hundreds and probably even thousands of antioxidants, most of them found naturally in plants, particularly fresh fruits and vegetables, but also in herbs. Antioxidants are also present to some degree in seafood, and in some animal foods.

Antioxidants neutralize the damage of oxidation by squelching free radicals. What does all that mean? We can think of oxidation as similar to what happens to metal when it rusts, or what happens to an apple when it turns brown. Have you ever prevented a cut-up apple from turning brown by squeezing some lemon juice on it? The vitamin C in the lemon juice is an antioxidant that is stopping the oxidation process. When meat spoils, or oil goes rancid, oxidation is in process.

An unstable oxygen molecule has a missing electron, creating what is called a free radical. These unstable oxygen molecules go to war in the body, grabbing onto other cells in their attempt to find another electron and stabilize. Every time a free radical stabilizes itself by attacking another cell, it leaves the cell it attacked damaged. That cell becomes unstable and in turn goes after another, creating a chain reaction. This is the process known as oxidation.

The damage free radicals do includes cell mutation, cardiovascular disease, cataracts, macular degeneration, arthritis, diseases affecting the brain, the kidneys, the lungs, the digestive system and the immune system. Free radicals are involved in the damage done by alcoholism, aging, radiation injury, iron overload, and diseases that affect the blood, such as strokes. Once the process of oxidation begins, it can be hard to stop, so your best health plan is to prevent it in the first place.

Our bodies naturally produce free radicals as part of our complex interaction with oxygen. In fact, free radicals act as enzymes and chemical messengers, and we couldn't live without them. It is when they become excessive that we begin to get sick. They have become a problem largely because of the polluted environment we live in, and our poor diets.

The ideal body, with ideal nutrition, in an ideal environment, would have the ability to counteract the free radicals it produces with the antioxidants it takes in and produces, and keep them under control. Heavy exercise produces free radicals, but it also has beneficial effects on the body that help counteract them.

Every day we encounter dozens of environmental causes of free radical production. The biggest culprits we know of are pollutants such as smog, toxins such as chlorine, herbicides and pesticides, radiation, some food additives, cigarette smoke, many prescription drugs, and rancid oil. Furthermore, most Americans eat relatively few fresh fruits and vegetables, one of our main natural sources of antioxidants. In a typical day, most of us run into more free radical-producing situations than our bodies can keep up with. This is why we need antioxidant supplements.

Let's take a quick look at some of my favorite antioxidants.

COENZYME Q10 (UBIQUINOL)

This versatile and powerful antioxidant is the superstar when it comes to fighting "bad" or LDL cholesterol. It works well in combination with vitamin E.

CoQ10 is a vital enzyme, or catalyst to the production of energy in our cells. Without it, our cells simply won't work. Its chemical name is *ubiquinone*—it is ubiquitous, or everywhere, where there is life. Its levels in the human body are highest in the heart and liver. When we are ill or stressed, and as we age, our bodies are less able to produce CoQ10.

CoQ10 helps regulate heart function. Many older people whose heart function has degenerated and who try CoQ10, report an almost immediate boost in their energy levels. People who suffer from angina report that the pain disappears and they can do some exercise. Studies have shown that people on heart medications can greatly reduce their dosage of medicine if it is combined with CoQ10.

CoQ10 can work powerfully to heal gum disease.

Food sources are mackerel, sardines, soybeans, peanuts and walnuts.

All CoQ10 is not created equal—the powder inside the capsules should be dark yellow.

SUPEROXIDE DISMUTASE (SOD)

Superoxide dismutase (SOD) is an enzyme that acts as a potent antioxidant, especially with skin tissue, and may be able to slow the aging process. SOD is destroyed in the stomach, so it needs to be used either as a cream or taken in an enteric coated capsule which passes through the stomach intact and dissolves in the intestines. SOD injections have been used successfully to treat scleroderma, a hardening of the skin. SOD with liposome is expensive, but if you have a stubborn skin problem it might be worth a try.

THE BIOFLAVONOID ANTIOXIDANTS

QUERCETIN

You should get to know this antioxidant, anticancer and antiallergy agent. This bioflavonoid may also have antiviral properties. Red and yellow onions are the best food sources of quercetin, though most fruits and vegetables contain some. You can also get it as a supplement.

PROANTHOCYANIDINS/PCOS/GRAPESEED EXTRACT

PCOs are another powerful free radical neutralizer that, like quercetin, are a bioflavonoid. Because PCOs are water soluble, the body is able to quickly and easily use them as an antioxidant. They also reduce inflammation, improve circulation, and improve the flexibility of connective tissues. Although proanthocyanidins are found in many fruits and vegetables, much of the supply is depleted by the time it gets to our stomachs. Most fruits and vegetables are grown in depleted soil, picked before they are ripened, sprayed with pesticides and fungicides, and stored for long periods of time.

PCOs can also be very effective in relieving allergy symptoms, because they inhibit the release of histamines.

GINKGO BILOBA

Ginkgo biloba has been used by the Chinese medicinally for at least 5,000 years. They prize ginkgo leaves for their ability to improve blood flow to the brain, open up congested lungs, and improve blood flow to the extremities. The leaves of this ancient tree provide a powerful antiaging aid, particularly in regard to improving brain function. It improves memory, learning and communication ability, as well as other symptoms of senility. It can also cure dizziness and improve balance.

Ginkgo is one of the best-selling medicines in Europe, sold to an estimated 10 million people every year. It has been the subject of over 300 scientific studies. GBE, a standardized ginkgo biloba extract, is a government-approved medicine in Germany and is covered by health insurance there.

Ginkgo's healing abilities have to do with improving circulation and improving the flow of oxygen to the brain and extremities. However, its spectrum of activities is wide, thanks to the wide variety of substances it contains, including flavonoids, terpenoids (ginkgolides, bilobalide), ginkgo heterosides, proanthocyanidins (PCO's) and organic acids.

Ginkgo is also useful for treating vision problems such as cataracts, macular degeneration, varicose veins, cold or numb feet and hands, ringing of the ears (tinnitus), leg cramps, and headaches. It improves cholesterol levels and improves circulation to the heart.

GREEN TEA

Green tea, the most popular of Asian drinks, turns out to be a potent antioxidant. The antioxidants specific to green tea are polyphenols, bioflavonoids that act as super antioxidants by neutralizing harmful fats and oils, lowering cholesterol and blood pressure, blocking cancer-triggering mechanisms, inhibiting bacteria and viruses, improving digestion, and protecting against ulcers and strokes. The specific type of polyphenol found in green tea is called a catechin.

Green tea comes from the same plants as black tea does, but is simply picked and dried without fermentation, allowing more of the original catechin content to remain intact. Oolong, a semi-fermented tea, falls in between black and green tea. Green tea contains 30-42 percent catechins, Oolong tea contains 8-20 percent catechins, and black tea contains 3-10 percent catechins.

CHAPTER 6

The Wonder of Enzymes

There isn't a cell in the body that functions without the help of enzymes. Enzymes are the magic ingredient that makes all of the other ingredients in the body work together. It is estimated that enzymes are facilitating 36 million biochemical reactions in the human body every minute. There are thousands of different enzymes at work, each with its own individual assignment.

Without the appropriate enzyme to bind to, vitamins are just so much organic matter, minerals are just so much inorganic matter, and even oxygen itself is just another molecule. Enzymes regulate all living matter, plants and animals alike. Take away enzymes and you no longer have something that is living.

We can also look at enzymes as the guide that shows the vitamin or mineral or fat the way into the cell. Without the introduction of the enzyme, the cell might never know the identity of the nutrient. Enzymes also speed up processes which might take much longer without their help, they build proteins that create tissue, remove toxins, help prevent the aging process within cells, and change nutrients into useful energy.

The enzymes that we know about are divided by what their purpose is in the body: they are called oxidoreductases, transferases, hydrolases, lyases, isomerases, and ligases. The digestive enzymes are the hydrolases, and these are the ones we will examine more closely.

We are born with enzymes already in our bodies, and we get some from food. However, enzymes are very sensitive to heat and processing, (including microwaving and pasteurizing) so they are not found in cooked or processed food. This means you need to get your enzymes from fresh, uncooked food such as raw fruit and vegetables, or from enzyme supplements.

Some enzyme experts believe that factors such as stress, malnutrition, junk food, alcohol and cigarettes destroy and thus deplete enzymes. They theorize that many digestive problems and immune disorders happen when we are deficient in enzymes.

Some of the best food sources of enzymes are avocados, bananas, papayas, mangoes, pineapples, sprouts and the aspergillus plant.

ENZYMES AND PAIN

There are new clinical studies showing that enzymes help reduce inflammation caused by arthritis, injuries to joints and other connective tissues such as muscle sprains, and can even relieve back pain. Enzymes tend to speed up the rate at which many bodily processes work, and injuries are no exception. Enzymes working at the site of an injury go to work to remove damaged tissue, which reduces swelling, and to help the body repair itself. As the enzymes do their work, they also become an effective pain reliever. The enzymes trypsin, chymotrypsin, papain and bromelain have been most commonly used in the studies involving enzymes and pain relief.

THE DIGESTIVE ENZYMES—NATURE'S WONDER WORKERS

Most enzymes are extremely tiny and found in very small quantities in the body. They work in organs, blood and tissue. The digestive enzymes, however, are a different story. Although you still need a microscope to see them, they are much larger than most other enzymes, and are present in the digestive system in large amounts. Since each digestive enzyme works with a specific food, a shortage or absence of even a single enzyme can make all the difference between health and sickness.

Enzymes are the catalysts in the digestive process. Food only becomes useful to the body after it has been converted to its component carbohydrates, proteins and fats in the digestive process. Only after digestion can valuable vitamins, minerals and amino acids be released and absorbed to keep us alive and healthy. The digestive enzymes cause biological reactions in our digestive systems without themselves being changed.

Each digestive enzyme works on a specific food type to break it down for absorption. One enzyme cannot substitute for another or do another's work. Enzymes that end in -ase are named by the food substance they act upon. For example, the enzyme that acts on phosphorus is named phosphatase; one of the enzymes that works on sugar (sucrose) is called sucrase.

As nutrients move through the digestive system and into the cells, they are helped along in the process by at least one enzyme. Although an enzyme is a protein, in order for it to work properly, it needs an amino acid and a coenzyme. Most coenzymes are vitamins and minerals. Two of the most important mineral coenzymes are magnesium and zinc. Magnesium alone is an essential co-factor (meaning it won't work without the magnesium present) for more than 300 different enzymes. Other minerals include iron, copper, manganese, selenium and molybdenum. The B vitamins thiamin, riboflavin, pantothenic acid and biotin are all coenzymes that help us digest starches, fats and proteins.

There are four known categories of digestive or hydrolytic enzymes:

1. **Amylase** or **amylolytic enzymes** are found in the saliva, pancreas, and intestines. They aid in the breakdown of carbohydrates.

2. **Protease** or **proteolytic enzymes** are found in the stomach, pancreas and intestines. They aid in the breakdown of proteins.

3. **Lipase** or **lipolytic enzymes** aid in the breakdown of fats.

4. **Cellulase** aids in breaking down cellulose.

AMYLASE ENZYMES THAT DIGEST STARCHES

Alpha-amylase is found in saliva and in the pancreas. It helps break down starches into sugars.

Beta-amylase is found in raw, unprocessed grains and vegetables, and also helps break down starch to sugar.

Mylase and **glucomylase** are starch-digesting enzymes capable of dissolving thousands of times their own weight in starches in the small intestine.

PROTEASE ENZYMES THAT DIGEST PROTEINS

Prolase is a concentrated protein-digesting enzyme derived from papain, which is extracted from papaya.

Protease is also extracted from papaya.

Bromelain is a digestive enzyme derived from pineapple.

Pepsin is released in the stomach, and splits protein into amino acids. In supplements, pepsin is made from animal enzymes.

Trypsin and **chymotrypsin,** produced by the pancreas, break down proteins.

Renin causes milk to coagulate, changing its protein, casein, into a form the body can use. Renin also releases minerals from milk, such as calcium, phosphorus, potassium and iron.

Pancreatin is an enzyme derived from the sections of an animal pancreas. This enzyme functions best in the small intestine.

HOW LIPASE WORKS

The efficient breakdown of fats plays a critical role in our health. Lipase and phospholipase act to break down fats in many stages, beginning with the upper portion of the stomach, called the cardial region. Here the lipase enzymes work in the acidic environment of the stomach to produce specific breakdown substances. If we aren't supplying enough enzymes here and in the main portion of the stomach to break down the fat we eat, when it reaches the small intestines it puts a much bigger load on the pancreas. The lipases supplied by the pancreas only work in the alkalinity of the small intestines, producing a whole different set of fat breakdown products than the acidic environment of the stomach. An enzyme supplement can greatly aid the digestive system by making sure that fats we eat are well down the road to digestion by the time they reach the small intestine.

HOW TO TAKE DIGESTIVE ENZYMES

When you take a digestive enzyme, be sure to take one that includes the three major types of enzymes: amylase, protease (or proteolytic enzymes) and lipase. If you eat dairy products and want some help digesting the lactose in them, get an enzyme supplement that contains lactase. Take them just before or with meals.

CHAPTER 7

How Drugs Can Deplete Nutrients

In North America we are addicted to drugs, and I don't mean the street drugs. It would probably be more accurate to say that our doctors and our mainstream medical system are addicted to drugs. The medical mind set is to diagnose a disease and then prescribe a pill for it. Very little thought is given to what caused the disease in the first place, or whether lifestyle changes and nutrition could correct the disease. As a result, Americans, and particularly older Americans, are, on the average, taking from three to eight drugs.

I call this the drug treadmill. You go to get a physical checkup with your doctor after the age of 50, and if you have slightly high cholesterol or blood pressure, if your joints hurt, or if your blood sugar is a bit off balance, you're likely to be put on a drug, with no suggestion that dietary changes or exercise might help. That drug will cause side effects. When you complain of these side effects to your doctor, you will be prescribed another drug, which in turn will cause a new set of side effects, for which you will be prescribed yet another drug, and so on. Pretty soon you're feeling tired all the time, you're depressed, gaining weight, can't sleep, have a chronic cough and no sex drive. You're not exercising any more and you're drinking twice as much coffee and eating twice as much sugar to try to bring your energy up. If you complain to your doctor about all the drugs and all the side effects, you will be threatened with the dire consequences of going off the drugs and told the side effects are simply part of old age. Hogwash!

First, I want you to know that nearly all the diseases of old age can be very well managed naturally with herbs and supplements that have few or no side effects. And most of these ailments can be prevented or reversed simply by lifestyle changes that include drinking plenty of fresh, clean water, getting some moderate exercise, cutting down on fat (particularly the hydrogenated oils) and sugar, eating plenty of fresh vegetables and taking some supplements. There is no reason why the vast majority of us can't enjoy a relatively pain-free old age with energy and vigor.

Nearly all the prescription and over-the-counter drugs prescribed by your doctor will have side effects. In the following pages I am going to list some nutrients that are depleted by some of the more common drugs. But I want you to educate yourself. There are many books available now on prescription drugs that can be understood by the average person. Read up on the drugs you're taking to find out if they are really safe and effective and what the side effects are. And even more important, take the steps to get off the drugs (with your doctor's guidance please) and take care of yourself.

Many prescription drugs cause depletion of the body's essential vitamins and minerals. A recent scientific study shows that ingredients found in common over-the-counter (OTC) cold, pain and allergy remedies actually lower the blood level of vitamin A in animals. Because vitamin A protects and strengthens the mucous membranes lining the nose, throat and lungs, a deficiency of vitamin A could actually break down these membranes, giving bacteria a cozy home to multiply in. Therefore, the drugs that are supposed to alleviate the cold may be actually prolonging it!

ASPIRIN

Aspirin is being touted as the new wonder drug to take for everything from heart disease to colon cancer. These claims are very flimsy and based more on advertising than on reality. You should know that 4,000 people die from the side effects of aspirin every year, and an additional 60,000 are hospitalized. Aspirin is well-known for causing gastrointestinal bleeding, and even a small amount of aspirin can *triple* the excretion rate of vitamin C from the body. In addition, aspirin can contribute to a deficiency of folic acid, one of the B vitamins. A deficiency of folic acid can lead to anemia, digestive disturbances, graying hair and growth problems. Taking aspirin at night will reduce the production of the hormone melatonin, and may result in insomnia.

CORTICOSTEROIDS

In spite of their horrendous side effects if used long-term, including bone loss and fragile skin, millions of people are dependent on corticosteroids such as Prednisone. These belong to a class of drugs called cortisones, used to ease the pain of arthritis, relieve lung congestion, and treat autoimmune diseases. They are also prescribed for skin problems and blood and eye disorders. Researchers conducted a study of 24 asthmatics using cortisone-type drugs and found the zinc levels were 42 percent lower than in patients not treated with corticosteroids. A zinc deficiency can lead to loss of taste and smell as well as a loss in sexual desire. Zinc is necessary for male potency and the health of the prostate gland. Zinc also enhances wound healing and is essential for a clear complexion.

BIRTH CONTROL PILLS

Oral contraceptives are made from a synthetic hormone that can lead to a deficiency of zinc, folic acid, vitamins C, B_6 and B_{12}. Deficiency of B_{12} can lead to emotional mood swings. B_6 deficiency can cause depression (many women on the pill are depressed). Women taking oral contraceptives (birth control pills) should take at least an extra 25-50 mg of B_6, 1,000 mcg of B_{12}, 400 mg of folic acid and 1,000 mg of vitamin C. Low vitamin C levels may account for increased susceptibility to blood clotting. I would recommend that you use another method of birth control, as the Pill raises your risk of strokes and cancer and causes many unpleasant side effects.

ANTACIDS

Antacids are routinely prescribed for digestive complaints such as heartburn or ulcers. In truth, what most people need is to cut back on the coffee, sugar, fatty, greasy and spicy foods, eat less, and to exercise more. Antacids interfere with the proper absorption of nutrients. Antacids that contain aluminum disturb calcium and phosphorus metabolism. Phosphorus deficiency, which is very rare (except in antacid users), can cause fatigue, loss of appetite and fragile bones.

DIURETICS

Diuretics, which are commonly prescribed for high blood pressure, also flush potassium and other minerals out of the body. Even potassium-sparing diuretics do not spare other minerals. You should be doubling your intake of minerals if you're taking diuretics.

PART II
Putting Together Your
Personal Vitamin Plan

CHAPTER 8

My Basic Adult Vitamin-Mineral Program

Not everyone requires the same vitamins/minerals. But here is my basic program, which you can then adapt according to the guidelines in the following pages for specific ages and problems. There are many multiple vitamins available that will give you the dosages listed below. Look for one that dissolves easily, is small enough to swallow easily, that uses natural not synthetic vitamins, and that doesn't use binders, fillers or colorings.

Ideally you'll take a high-potency multiple vitamin at least twice a day that gives you:

Beta-carotene or carotenoids, 10,000-15,000 IU

The B vitamins, including:
B_1 (thiamine), 25-50 mg
B_2 (riboflavin), 25-100 mg
B_3 (niacin), 25-100 mg
B_5 (pantothenic acid), 25-100 mg
B_6 (pyridoxine), 50-100 mg
B_{12} (cobalamin) 100-1,000 mcg
Biotin, 100-300 mcg
Choline, 25-100 mg
Folic acid, 200-400 mcg
Inositol, 100-300 mg

Vitamin D, 100-500 IU

Vitamin C, 1000-3000 mg

Vitamin E, at least 400 IU

Minerals
  Boron, 1-5 mg
  Calcium (citrate, lactate or gluconate), 100-500 mg
    (women should take a total of 600-1,200 mg daily)
  Chromium (picolinate), 200-400 mcg
  Copper, 1-5 mg
  Magnesium (citrate or gluconate), 100-500 mg (women
    should take a total of 300-600 mg daily)
  Manganese (citrate or chelate), 10 mg
  Selenium, 25-50 mcg
  Vanadium (vanadyl sulfate), 25-200 mcg
  Zinc, 10-15 mg

Since vitamin C, vitamin E, calcium and magnesium tend to make a multivitamin pill larger, you can take a multivitamin with smaller amounts of those vitamins and then take the others separately. A calcium/magnesium combination works well at bedtime when it will help you relax and prevent leg cramps.

CHAPTER 9

Vitamins for Children

Children's nutritional needs are different from adults not only because they're growing, but also because they're smaller.

Your doctor can recommend liquid vitamins for infants and toddlers. If you are vegetarian, I recommend an additional amino acid supplement that includes all of the essential amino acids plus histidine, taurine and cysteine, which are essential for growing children.

Here are recommendations for children from the age of four to pre-puberty, around the age of 11-13.

Vitamin A/beta-carotene   500-1,000 IU

The B vitamins, including:
   B_1 (thiamine), .9-1.3 mg
   B_2 (riboflavin), 1.1-1.5 mg
   B_3 (niacin), 12-17 mg
   B_5 (pantothenic acid), 4-50 mg
   B_6 (pyridoxine), 1.1-2 mg
   B_{12} (cobalamin), 3-5 mcg
   Biotin, 50-150 mcg
   Folic acid, 150-350 mcg

Vitamin D, 100 IU

Vitamin C, 150-500 mg

Vitamin E, 15-25 IU

Minerals

Calcium (citrate, lactate or gluconate), 800 mg

Chromium (picolinate), 80-200 mcg

Iron, 10-12 mg

Magnesium (citrate or gluconate), 200-300 mg

Selenium, 100-200 mcg

Zinc, 10 mg

Bioflavonoids (amount varies with the type, but they will enhance the action of the rest of the vitamins)

CHAPTER 10

Vitamins for Teens

Minimizing the consumption of junk food, maximizing the consumption of vegetables, and daily aerobic exercise is the best health program a teen can follow. Plenty of clean water will play a major role in preventing acne and clearing the body of toxins.

CALCIUM AND BONES

Please be sure they are getting enough calcium, as good bone growth in the teens can prevent osteoporosis later in life. A diet with too much protein (more than 2 ounces per day), and too many sodas containing phosphorus will leach calcium from the bones and can be the cause of osteoporosis later in life. Milk is not a very good source of calcium, because it has a poor calcium to magnesium ratio, and the bone building doesn't happen without magnesium. If your teens are milk drinkers, please have them take a magnesium tablet with their milk. Fresh vegetables are a much better source of calcium. Exercise is also one of the best ways to build strong bones, and will help balance the surges of hormones teens have to cope with.

ACNE

If your teens are having problems with acne, you can add a vitamin A supplement, 5,000 IU, an additional 400 IU of vitamin E, and a B-complex vitamin until it clears up. Avoiding refined carbohydrates such as cakes and cookies and fried foods will help tremendously. Yogurt is the best acne-prevention food a teen can eat, and will also supply calcium. Buy plain yogurt and sweeten it with fruit.

DEPRESSION

If your teen is suffering from depression, try a B-complex vitamin and some exercise.

BASIC RECOMMENDATIONS

Vitamin A/beta-carotene   5,000 IU

The B vitamins, including:
B_1 (thiamine), 1.5 mg
B_2 (riboflavin), 2 mg
B_3 (niacin), 18 mg
B_5 (pantothenic acid), 50 mg
B_6 (pyridoxine), 2.5 mg
B_{12} (cobalamin), 5 mcg
Biotin, 75-150 mcg
Folic acid, 200 mcg

Vitamin D, 100 IU

Vitamin C, 300-500 mg

Vitamin E, 50-100 IU

Minerals
Calcium (citrate, lactate or gluconate), 1,200 mg
Chromium (picolinate), 200 mcg
Iron, 18 mg
Magnesium (citrate or gluconate), 350-400 mg
Selenium, 200 mcg
Zinc, 10-15 mg

CHAPTER 11

Vitamins for Athletes

Athletes have special vitamin needs, as their metabolism tends to be higher than average, creating a greater need for some vitamins. In addition, exercise creates free radicals, so extra protection is needed. Please be sure to drink at least 8-10 glasses of clean water every day.

Here are some guidelines for athletes:

ANTIOXIDANT PROTECTION

Take an extra antioxidant supplement containing vitamin C, vitamin E, beta carotene, selenium, and a bioflavonoid antioxidant such as green tea extract, PCO's (grapeseed extract), rutin, hesperidin, quercetin, or a combination.

OPTIMAL HEALING

To speed healing of tissue and tendon injuries, in addition to the Basic Program for Adults, take:

Vitamin C 1,000 to 3,000 mg in divided doses, daily
Calcium pantothenate (vitamin B_5), 100 mg, 1-2 times daily
Vitamin B complex, 50 mg, twice daily
Vitamin D, 400 IU daily
Glucosamine sulfate (follow instructions on the bottle)
Ginkgo biloba

WEIGHT REDUCTION

Athletes who are trying to reduce their weight can take the following nutrients to enhance fat burning:

Chromium picolinate, 200 mcg daily
Carnitine (L-carnitine or N-acetyl carnitine), 500 mg once daily
Phenylalanine, 200-500 mg daily, ½ between meals, with water (Not to be used by anyone with PKU, skin cancer or high blood pressure. If you get headaches or dizziness, stop taking it.)

WEIGHT GAIN

The best key to weight gain is to shun the sugar and junk food and go for nutrition-packed foods such as avocados, nuts and seeds, sweet potatoes, dates, raisins and moderate amounts of cheese.

Vitamins that can improve appetite include:
Vitamin B-complex, 50 mg
Vitamin B_{12}, sublingual or intranasal

CHAPTER 12

Vitamins for Women

Women can have special vitamin needs depending on age and hormone balance.

PMS

There is no single solution or easy answer to premenstrual syndrome (PMS), because each woman who suffers from it may have a variety of symptoms and causes. However, there are a few things women can try that help nearly all women with PMS to some extent.

The first thing to try is a healthy diet and exercise: cut way back on refined sugars and carbohydrates, eliminate fried foods, emphasize whole grains and fresh vegetables, eat plenty of legumes, including soy products, and drink plenty of clean water.

If that doesn't work, try the supplements listed below, and if that doesn't work, try some natural progesterone cream. (See "Osteoporosis" below for details on natural progesterone).

In addition to the Basic Adult Program, daily vitamins for PMS include the following. They can either be taken premenstrually or throughout the month.

Vitamin B_6, 100-300 mg daily
Beta-carotene, 15,000 to 20,000 IU daily in divided doses
Choline, 500 mg
Inositol, 500 mg

Vitamin C, 1,000 mg
Vitamin E, 400 IU
Magnesium, 300 mg

PREMENOPAUSE

Many women today are suffering from "premenopause syndrome," caused by anovulatory (not ovulat-
ing) menstrual cycles in which no progesterone is
made, creating a relative excess of estrogen. The symptoms of premenopause syndrome include weight gain,
bloating, mood swings, cold hands and feet, irritability, unstable blood sugar, fatigue, and depression. The
treatment is the same as for PMS, and may require
extra support to the adrenal glands. For a detailed
explanation of premenopause syndrome and other
women's hormone balance issues, I highly recommend the book *What Your Doctor May Not Tell You About
Menopause: The Breakthrough Book on Natural Progesterone*, by John R. Lee, M.D. (Warner Books, 1996).

OSTEOPOROSIS

It is especially important that all women get enough
calcium to prevent osteoporosis, preferably through
fresh vegetables, especially the leafy green ones.
Women who drink a lot of phosphorus-containing
sodas and eat too much protein (more than 1.5
ounces per day) will lose calcium from their bones
regardless of how much calcium they take. Please eat
a plant-based diet with plenty of soy foods and strictly
limit your intake of sodas. It is also important to get
weight-bearing exercise, which builds bone.

I also recommend that all menopausal women at
risk for osteoporosis use a natural progesterone
cream, which actually stimulates bone building and
can reverse osteoporosis as well as prevent it. Estrogen

(such as Premarin) only slows bone loss for a few years around the time of menopause and creates a high risk of cancer, so for most women I don't recommend it. Natural progesterone has no known side effects and may actually be protective against breast cancer.

By "natural progesterone cream" I don't mean the synthetic progestins such as Provera, nor do I mean the "wild yam extract" creams containing diosgenin, a laboratory precursor of progesterone. To confuse matters even further, both the creams containing natural progesterone and those containing diosgenin may be labeled "wild yam extract." Your best bet is to use a reputable source. I recommend that to find out more about how to order and use natural progesterone cream, call Professional Technical Services in Eugene, Oregon at 1-800-888-6814.

Women at risk for osteoporosis should take the following supplements, in addition to the Basic Adult Program:

Vitamin B$_6$, 50 mg/day
Calcium/magnesium, 600 mg calcium/300 mg magnesium

MENOPAUSE

Menopausal women are at higher risk of heart disease and osteoporosis, but I promise you, estrogen is not the solution! After an initial period of feeling better, estrogen and the synthetic progestins cause most women to feel as if they have permanent PMS! The not-found-in-nature synthetic hormones prescribed by most doctors do vastly more harm than good, and their ability to protect against heart disease and osteoporosis is grossly exaggerated by pharmaceutical companies eager to cash in on the discomfort of millions of menopausal women.

The problems associated with menopause are also grossly exaggerated by the drug companies and the media. In truth, it is women who have had a hysterectomy (instant menopause) who have the most problems. The vast majority of other women pass through menopause relatively uneventfully.

Your best bet for preventing and relieving menopause symptoms such as hot flashes and vaginal dryness is plenty of exercise, clean water and a nutrition-rich, low-fat diet emphasizing vegetables and soy products. Menopause symptoms are virtually nonexistent in Japan, where fat consumption is low and soy consumption is high.

Any woman with the menopause symptoms listed above and/or hair loss, dry skin, and decreased libido not relieved by the above lifestyle guidelines plus the vitamins below, should try natural progesterone cream. (See the section on osteoporosis for more information on natural progesterone.) Any woman at risk for heart disease or osteoporosis should also be using natural progesterone cream. Recent research indicates that natural progesterone may also be protective against breast cancer.

In addition to the Basic Adult Program, vitamins for women with menopause symptoms should include:

Vitamin B_6, 100-300 mg daily
Beta-carotene, 15,000 to 20,000 IU daily in divided
    doses
Choline, 500 mg
Inositol, 500 mg
Vitamin C, 1,000 mg
Vitamin E, 400 IU
Magnesium, 300 mg

CHAPTER 13

Vitamins for Pregnant Women

Pregnant women have special vitamin needs both to support the growing fetus and to support themselves. There are also supplements to avoid when you are pregnant. The best rule of thumb when considering whether to take any type of supplement, pill or potion when pregnant is: when in doubt, don't.

And remember, no vitamin regimen is a substitute for a balanced diet of wholesome foods including whole grains, fresh fruits and vegetables, legumes, and moderate amounts of protein.

The Basic Adult Program will work well with pregnancy, with the following changes and cautions:

Folic acid is an extremely important vitamin in preventing birth defects such as neural tube defects (spina bifida). Women of child-bearing age who are at any risk of getting pregnant should be taking 400 mcg of folic acid daily.

Women experiencing morning sickness can take 30-50 mg of vitamin B_6, which should solve the problem.

If you are suffering from varicose veins or other signs of poor circulation in the extremities, you can take the recommended dose of a standardized ginkgo biloba extract.

Vitamins women should avoid during pregnancy include vitamin A (use beta carotene), and please don't overdo it on the iron—no more than 30 mg daily.

Pregnant women should take extra calcium and magnesium, 600 mg of calcium and 300 mg of magnesium, and extra zinc for a total of 25 mg. The calcium and magnesium should be taken separately from the iron, because they can interfere with iron absorption.

The problem of preeclampsia, also called toxemia, or pregnancy-induced high blood pressure, is nearly always caused by a magnesium deficiency. Your best bet is to prevent it by taking magnesium from day one.

A pregnancy multiple vitamin should contain all the essential minerals and the trace minerals chromium, manganese and molybdenum.

CHAPTER 14

Vitamins for Men

Men have special vitamin needs, mostly based on the fact of aging and declining hormone production. Men with an active sex life can also deplete vitamins E, selenium and zinc which are found in high concentrations in semen.

STRESS VITAMINS

Men who are under stress should take the following supplements daily, in addition to the Basic Adult Program:

Zinc, 15 mg
Selenium, 100 mcg
Vitamin B complex, 50 mg
Vitamin A, 5,000 IU
Vitamin C, 1,000 mg
Vitamin E, 400 IU

PROSTATE PROBLEMS

Men who have an enlarged prostate or are having symptoms of an enlarged prostate such as getting up repeatedly during the night to urinate, dribbling, and urgency, should take the following supplements in addition to the Basic Adult Program:

Zinc, 15 mg
Selenium, 100 mcg

Vitamin E, 400 IU
Vitamin B complex, 50 mg
Saw palmetto berries and pygeum extract (follow
   directions on the bottle)
Pumpkin seeds, eat a handful daily (unsalted, raw)

INCREASED SEX DRIVE

Supplements that can improve libido include:

Tyrosine, 250-500 mg daily
Phenylalanine, 250-500 mg daily
Vitamin A, 5,000 to 10,000 IU daily
Vitamin C, 1,000 mg daily
Siberian ginseng in tea, capsules or tincture
Lecithin (granules or capsules), be sure it's fresh
   and not rancid

CHAPTER 15

Vitamins for Seniors

As we age we have special vitamin needs for a variety of reasons. One is that the signals from the hypothalamus and pituitary glands that regulate hormones wane, and the other is that digestion and absorption of nutrients become less efficient, vastly decreasing the amount of nutrients taken in by the body, even with a good diet. This makes supplements especially important as part of an antiaging program.

Over and over again, studies have shown that eating plenty of fresh vegetables and moderate exercise are two of your keys to a healthy and energetic old age.

For more detail on the foods, herbs and supplements that work to slow the aging process, I recommend my books, *Earl Mindell's Anti-Aging Bible* (Simon & Schuster, 1996) and *Dr. Earl Mindell's What You Should Know about the Super Antioxidant Miracle* (Keats Publishing, 1996).

Here are the extra supplements I recommend for seniors in addition to the Basic Adult Program:

Glucosamine sulfate (for stiff joints), follow directions on bottle

Betaine hydrochloride (to aid digestion), follow directions on bottle

Digestive enzymes (follow directions on bottle)

Vitamin B_{12}, 1,000 mg every three days, sublingually or intranasally

Vitamin B_6, 50 mg daily

Folic acid, 100 mcg daily

Bioflavonoid antioxidant formula (for example, rutin, hesperidin, PCO's as grapeseed extract, green tea extract, quercetin)

Ginkgo biloba (follow directions on the bottle)

Melatonin (if you're having trouble sleeping), 1.5 mg 1 hour before bed

Magnesium, 300 mg daily

Glutathione (take N-acetyl cysteine, a precursor), follow directions on bottle

Coenzyme Q10, 30-90 mg daily

L-carnitine, 500-1,000 mg daily

Ginseng (when recovering from illness or for stamina)

GLOSSARY

absorption The process by which nutrients are passed into the bloodstream.

acetate A derivative of **acetic acid.**

acetic acid Used as a synthetic flavoring agent, one of the first food additives (vinegar is approximately 4 to 6 per cent acetic acid); it is found naturally in cheese, coffee, grapes, peaches, raspberries and strawberries. Generally Recognized As Safe **(GRAS)** when used only in packaging.

acetylcholine One of the chemicals involved in the transmission of nerve impulses.

adrenalin(e) A hormone secreted by the **adrenal glands** into the bloodstream in response to physical or mental stress, such as fear or injury; works with **noradrenalin(e)** to regulate blood pressure and heart rate.

adrenal glands The glands, located above each kidney, that manufacture **adrenalin(e), noradrenalin(e),** and **steroids.**

aldosterone A hormone secreted by the **adrenal glands** which regulates the salt and water balance in the body; one of the **steroids.**

alkaline Containing an acid-neutralizing substance (being alkaline, sodium bicarbonate is used for excess acidity in foods).

allergen A substance that causes an **allergy.**

amino acid chelates Chelated minerals that have been produced by many of the same processes nature uses to **chelate** minerals in the body; in the digestive tract, nature surrounds the elemental minerals with **amino acid,** permitting them to be absorbed into the bloodstream.

amino acids The organic compounds from which proteins are constructed; 22 amino acids have been identified as necessary to the human body; 9 are known as essential—histidine, isoleucine, leucine, lysine, total S-containing amino acids, total aromatic amino acids, threonine, tryptophan, and valine—and must be obtained from food.

amenorrhea Absence or suppression of menstruation.

androgen Any of the group of hormones which stimulates male characteristics.

angina pectoris A cramping pain in the chest, stemming from the heart and often spreading to the left shoulder and arm.

anorexia Loss of appetite, especially resulting from disease.

anorexia nervosa A psychophysiological disorder featuring an abnormal fear of becoming obese, a persistent aversion to food, a distorted self-image, and severe loss of weight.

antibody A protein substance produced in the blood or tissues in response to a specific **antigen,** such as a **toxin** or bacteria; by neutralizing **organic** poisons and weakening or destroying bacteria, antibodies form the basis of immunity.

antigen Any substance not normally present in the body that stimulates the body to produce antibodies.

antihistamine A drug used to reduce effects associated with **histamine** production in allergies and colds.

antineoplastics Drugs that prevent the growth and development of malignant cells.

antioxidant A substance that can protect another substance from **oxidation**; added to foods to keep oxygen from changing the food's color.

antitoxin An **antibody** formed in response to, and capable of neutralizing, a poison of biological origin.

arthritis Inflammation of joints.

arteriosclerosis A disease of the arteries characterized by hardening, thickening, and loss of elasticity of the arterial walls; results in impaired blood circulation.

assimilation The process whereby nutrients are used by the body and changed into living tissue.

asthma A condition of lungs characterized by a decrease in diameter of some air passages; a spasm of the bronchial tubes or swelling of their mucous membranes.

ataxia Loss of coordinated movement caused by disease of the nervous system.

atherosclerosis A process where fatty deposits in the walls of arteries make the walls thick and hard, narrowing the arteries; a form of **arteriosclerosis**.

ATP A molecule called adenosine triphosphate, the fuel of life, a nucleotide—building block of **nucleic acid**—that produces biological energy with vitamins B_1, B_2, B_3, and pantothenic acid, another B complex **vitamin**.

autoimmunity An abnormal condition where the body produces antibodies against its own tissues.

avidin A protein in egg white capable of inactivating **biotin**.

bacteriophage A **virus** that infects bacteria.

basal metabolic rate The body's rate of metabolism when at rest.

basophil A type of white blood cell representing less than 1% of the total.

B cells White blood cells, made in bone marrow, which produce antibodies upon instructions from T cells, manufactured in the **thymus**.

beta-carotene A plant pigment which can be converted into two forms of **vitamin** A.

BHA Butylated hydroxyanisole; a preservative and **antioxidant** used in many products; insoluble in water; can be toxic to the kidneys.

BHT Butylated hydroxytoluene; a solid, white crystalline **antioxidant** used to retard spoilage of many foods; can be more toxic to the kidney than its nearly identical chemical cousin, **BHA.**

bioflavonoids A group of compounds needed to maintain healthy blood vessel walls; found chiefly as coloring matter in flowers and fruits, particularly yellow ones; known as vitamin P complex.

biotin A colorless, crystalline B complex **vitamin**; essential for the activity of many **enzyme** systems; helps produce **fatty acids**; found in large quantities in liver, egg yolk, milk, and yeast.

bursa A pouch or sac containing fluid for the lubrication of joints.

bursitis Swelling or inflammation of a **bursa.**

calciferol A colorless, odorless crystalline material, insoluble in water; soluble in fats; a synthetic form of **vitamin** D made by irradiating **ergosterol** with ultraviolet light.

calcium gluconate An **organic** calcium based compound.

capillary A minute blood vessel, one of many that connect the arteries and veins and deliver oxygen to tissues.

carcinogen A cancer-causing substance.

cardiotonic A compound which aids the heart.

cardiovascular Relating to the heart and blood vessels.

carotene An orange-yellow pigment occuring in many plants and capable of being converted into **vitamin** A in the body.

casein The **protein** in milk that has become the standard by which protein quality is measured.

catabolism The metabolic change of nutrients or complex substances into simpler compounds, accompanied by a release of energy.

catalyst A substance that modifies, especially increases, the rate of chemical reaction without being consumed or changed in the process.

cellulose Carbohydrate found in the outer layers of fruits and vegetables which is undigestible.

cerebrovascular accident A blood clot or bleeding in the brain; a stroke.

chelation A process by which mineral substances are changed into an easily digestible form.

cholesterol A white, crystalline substance, made up of various fats; naturally produced in vertebrate animals and humans; important as a precursor to steroid hormones and as a constituent of cell membranes.

chronic Of long duration, continuing, constant.

CNS Central nervous system.

coenzyme A substance that combines with other substances to form a complete **enzyme**; nonprotein and usually a B **vitamin**.

collagen The primary **organic** constituent of bone, cartilage and connective tissue (becomes gelatin through boiling).

complex carbohydrate Fibrous molecules of starch or sugar which slowly release sugar into the bloodstream.

congenital Condition existing at birth, not hereditary.

coronary occlusion Blockage of a heart artery.

coronary thrombosis Blood clot in a heart artery.

corticosteroids See **steroids**.

dermatitis An inflammation of the skin; a rash.

diastolic Second number in a blood pressure reading; measures the pressure in arteries between contractions of the heart.

dicalcium phosphate A filler used in pills, which is derived from purified mineral rocks and is a source of calcium and phosphorus.

demineralization The loss of minerals or salts from bone and tissue.

diluents Fillers; inert material added to tablets to increase their bulk in order to make them a practical size for compression.

disaccharide A sugar which breaks down into two **monosaccharides**.

diuretic Tending to increase the flow of urine from the body.

DNA Deoxyribonucleic acid; the **nucleic acid** in chromosomes that is part of the chemical basis for hereditary characteristics.

emulsion A substance with chemical characteristics of both water and oil; aids mixing and dispersing between the two.

endocrine Producing secretions passed directly to the **lymph** or blood instead of into a duct; to do with the endocrine glands or the **hormones** they produce.

endogenous Being produced from within the body.

endorphins Natural opiates produced in the brain; pain suppressants.

enteric coated A tablet coated so that it dissolves in the intestine, not in the acid environment of the stomach.

enzyme A **protein** substance found in living cells that brings about chemical changes; necessary for digestion of food; compounds with names ending in -*ase*.

epinephrine See **adrenalin(e)**

ergosterol A **vitamin** D group **steroid**; originally found in ergot, a fungal disease of rye; also found in other fungi, yeast, and mushrooms; changed by ultraviolet light into vitamin D_2

excipient Any inert substance used as a dilutant or vehicle for a drug.

exogenous Being derived or developed from external causes.

fatty acid Acids produced by the breakdown of fats; essential fatty acids cannot be produced by the body and must be included in the diet.

FDA Food and Drug Administration.

fibrin An insoluble **protein** that forms the necessary fibrous network in the coagulation of blood. An excess of fibrinogen in the blood increases the risk of heart disease.

free radicals Highly reactive chemical fragments that can beneficially act as chemical messengers, but in excess produce an irritation of artery walls and start the arteriosclerotic process if antioxidants are not present.

fructose A natural sugar occurring in fruits and honey, called fruit sugar; often used as a preservative for foodstuffs and an intravenous nutrient.

galactosemia A hereditary disorder in which ingested milk becomes toxic.

gland An organ in the body where certain substances in the blood are seperated and converted into secretions for use in the body (such as hormones) or to be discharged from the body (such as sweat); nonsecreting structures similar to glands, like **lymph** nodes, are also known as glands.

glucose Blood sugar; a product of the body's **assimilation** of carbohydrates and a major source of energy.

glutamic acid An **amino acid** present in all complete proteins; also manufactured commercially from vegetable protein; used as a salt substitute and a flavor-intensifying agent.

glutamine An **amino acid** that constitutes, with **glucose**, the major nourishment used by the nervous system.

gluten A mixture of two proteins, gliadin and glutenin, present in wheat, rye, oats, and barley.

glycogen The body's chief form of stored carbohydrate, primarily in the liver; coverted to **glucose** when needed.

GRAS Generally Recognized as Safe; a list established by Congress to cover substances added to food.

HDL High-density lipoprotein; HDL is sometimes called "good" **cholesterol** because it is the body's major carrier of cholesterol to the liver for excretion in the bile.

hemoglobin Molecule necessary for the transport of oxygen by red blood cells; iron is an essential component.

hesperidin Part of the **vitamin** C complex.

histamine An **organic** compound of ammonia released by the body in allergic reactions.

holistic treatment Treatment of the whole person, rather than just parts or symptoms.

homeostasis The body's physiological equilibrium.

hormone A substance formed in **endocrine** organs and transported by body fluids to activate other specifically receptive organs, cells or tissues.

humectant A substance that is used to preserve the moisture content of materials.

hydrochloric acid An acid secreted in the stomach; a main part of gastric juice.

hydrolyzed Put into water-soluble form.

hydrolyzed protein chelate Water-soluble and chelated for easy **assimilation**.

hyperglycemia A condition caused by high blood sugar.

hypoglycemia A condition caused by abnormally low blood sugar.

ichthyosis A condition characterized by a scaliness on the outer layer of skin.

idiopathic A condition whose causes are not yet known.

immune Protected against disease.

infarction Localized tissue death due to lack of oxygen supply.

insulin A **hormone**, secreted by the pancreas, that helps regulate the **metabolism** of sugar in the body.

interferon Any of a group of proteins produced by cells in response to infection by a **virus**; prevents viral replication and can induce resistance to viral antigens.

IU International Units

lactose One of the sugars found in milk.

lactating Producing milk.

LDL Low-density lipoprotein; sometimes referred to as "bad" **cholesterol**, LDLs easily become **oxidized** and carry cholesterol through the bloodstream; studies show high levels can increase risk of coronary artery disease (CAD).

lecithin Any of a group of fats rich in phosphorus; essential for transforming fats in the body; rich sources include egg yolk, soybeans and corn.

linoleic acid One of the polyunsaturated fats; an essential **fatty acid**; a constituent of **lecithin**; known as **vitamin F**; indispendable for life, and must be obtained from foods.

lipid A fat or fatty substance.

lipofuscin A group of fats, plentiful in adult cells and associated with aging.

lipotropic Preventing abnormal or excessive accumulation of fat; lipotropin is a **hormone** which stimulates the conversion of stored fat to usable, liquid form.

lymph The almost clear fluid flowing through the lymphatic vessels; lymph nourishes tissue cells and returns waste matter to the bloodstream.

lymphocyte Any of the almost colorless cells produced in lymphoid tissue, as in the **lymph** nodes, spleen, thymus, and tonsils; lymphocytes make up between 22 and 28 percent of adult human white blood cells; primarily responsible for **antibody** production, lymphocytes include **B cells** and **T cells.**

megavitamin therapy Treatment of illness with massive amounts of vitamins.

metabolism The processes of physical and chemical change where food is synthesised into living matter until it is broken down into simpler substances or waste matter; energy is produced by these processes.

monosaccharide A simple sugar with one molecular unit such as **glucose.**

mucopolysaccharide Thick gelatinous material that is found in many places in the body; it glues cells together and lubricates joints.

naturopathy The use of herbs and other methods to stimulate the body's innate defenses without using drugs.

neuropathy Symptoms caused by abnormalities in sensory or motor nerves.

neurotransmitter A chemical substance which transmits or changes nerve impulses.

nitrites Used as fixatives in cured meats; can combine with natural stomach and food chemicals to cause dangerous cancer-causing agents called nitrosamines.

noradrenalin(e) A hormone produced in the **adrenal glands** that increases blood pressure by blood vessel narrowing without affecting the heart's output; works with **epinephrine**.

norepinephrine See **noradrenalin(e)**.

nucleic acid Any of a group of complex compounds which form a major part of **DNA** and **RNA**; found in all living cells and viruses.

oncologist Specialist in tumors; cancer specialist.

organic Describes any chemical containing carbon; or any food or supplement made with animal or vegetable fertilizers; or produced without synthetic fertilizers or pesticides and free from chemical injections or additives.

orthomolecular The right molecule used for the right treatment; doctors who practice preventive medicine and use vitamin therapies are known as orthomolecular physicians.

OSHA Occupational Safety and Health Administration.

oxalates Organic chemicals found in certain foods, especially spinach, which can combine with calcium to form calcium oxalate, an insoluble chemical the body cannot use.

oxidation The way in which certain types of altered oxygen molecules cause biochemical reactions; examples are browning of apples and rancidity in oil.

PABA Para-aminobenzoic acid; a member of the **vitamin** B complex.

palmitate Water-solubilized **vitamin** A.

peroxides Free radicals formed as by-products when oxygen reacts with molecules of fat.

phytoestrogen Any of a number of compounds found in plants which occupy estrogen receptors and may help protect the body from the negative effects of excess estrogen.

PKU (phenylketonuria) A hereditary disease caused by the lack of an **enzyme** needed to convert an essential **amino acid** (phenylalanine) into a form usable by the body; can cause mental retardation unless detected early.

placebo A substance which produces no pharmacological activity; one used instead of and alongside an active substance for comparison.

polysaccharide A molecule made up of many sugar molecules joined together.

polyunsaturated fats Highly nonsaturated fats from vegetable sources; can dissolve or absorb other substances.

precancerous lesion Tissue that is abnormal but not yet malignant.

predigested protein Protein that has been processed for fast **assimilation** and can go directly into the bloodstream.

prostaglandins Hormonelike substances that aid in regulation of the immune system.

protein A complex substance containing nitrogen which is essential to plant and animal cells; ingested proteins are changed to **amino acids** in the body.

provitamin A **vitamin** precursor; a chemical substance necessary to produce a **vitamin**.

PUFA Polyunsaturated **fatty acid**.

RDA Recommended Dietary Allowances as established by the Food and Nutrition Board, National Academy of Sciences, National Research Council.

retrovirus A class of viruses containing **RNA**.

riboflavin Vitamin B_2; part of the B vitamin complex; yellow, crystallike **coenzyme** involved in the breakdown of proteins, fats and carbohydrates; must be obtained from food.

ribonucleic acid (RNA) A constituent of all living cells and many viruses; its structure determines **protein** synthesis and genetic transmission.

rose hip A rich source of **vitamin** C; the nodule underneath the bud of a rose called a hip, in which the plant produces vitamin C.

rutin A substance often extracted from buckwheat; part of the **vitamin** C complex.

saturated fatty acids Usually solid at room temperature; higher proportions found in foods from animal sources.

sclerosis The hardening or thickening of a part of the body, such as an artery.

sequestrant A substance that absorbs some of the products of chemical reactions; it prevents changes that would affect flavor, texture, and color of food; used for water softening.

serotonin A **neurotransmitter** considered essential for sleep and concentration.

serum Any thin, watery fluid; especially the clear, sticky part of blood that remains after clotting.

simple carbohydrate Simple sugar molecules, such as **glucose**, which are rapidly absorbed by the bloodstream.

steroids Hormones produced by the **adrenal glands** that influence or control key functions of the body; formed from **cholesterol**; three major types influencing skin, muscle, fat, and **metabolism** of **glucose**, sexual functions and characteristics, and processing of minerals; used as drugs such as cortisone to suppress the immune system, reduce inflammation and to treat allergies.

syncope Brief loss of consciousness; fainting.

synergistic The way two or more substances produce an effect that neither alone could accomplish.

synthetic Produced artificially; not found in nature.

systemic Capable of spreading through the entire body.

systolic First number in a blood pressure reading; measures the pressure in arteries as the heart contracts.

T Cells White blood cells, manufactured in the **thymus**, which protect the body from bacteria, viruses, and cancer-causing agents, while controlling the production of **B cells** which produce antibodies, and unwanted production of potentially harmful **T cells**.

teratological Monstrous or abnormal formations in animals or plants.

thymus Major gland of the immune system situated behind the top of the breastbone; site of **T cell** production.

tocopherols The group of compounds (alpha, beta, delta, episilon, eta, gamma and zeta) that make **vitamin** E; obtained through vacuum distillation of edible vegetable oils.

toxicity The quality or condition of being poisonous, harmful, or destructive.

toxin An **organic** poison produced in living or dead organisms.

triglycerides Fatty substances in the blood.

unsaturated fatty acids Most often liquid at room temperature; primarily found in vegetable fats.

virus Any of a large group of minute organisms that can only reproduce in the cells of plants and animals.

vitamin Any of about fifteen natural compounds essential in small amounts as catalysts for processes in the body; most cannot be made by the body and must come from diet.

xerosis Skin condition of dryness, lacking moisture or oil; often resulting in a pattern of fine lines, scaling and itching.

yeast Single celled fungus that can cause infections in the body.

zyme A fermenting substance.

INDEX

The glossary pages (71–84) are not indexed.

Dr. Earl Mindell's

What You Should Know About...
series
in print or forthcoming